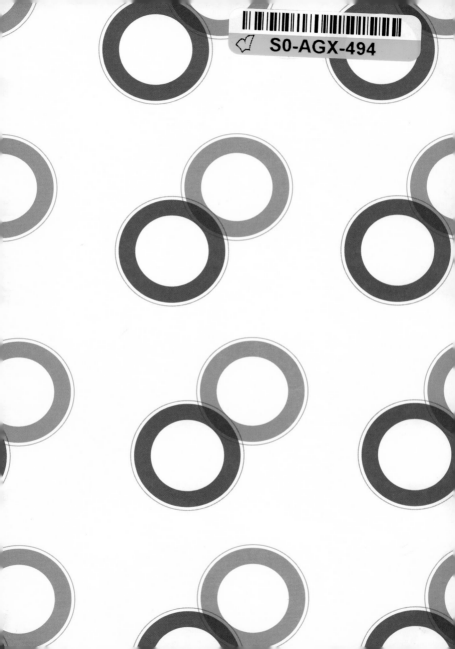

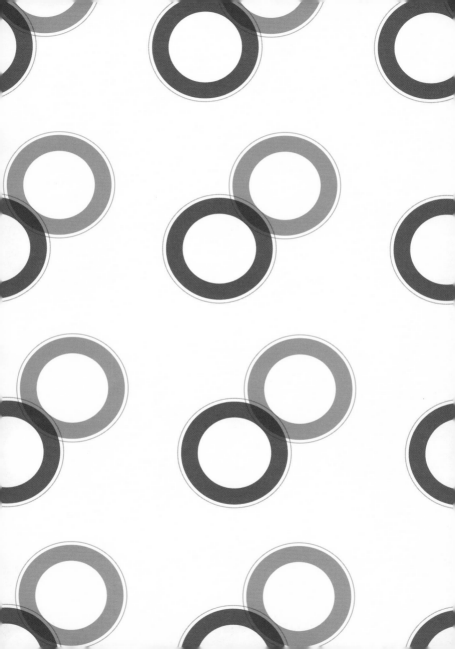

a **short guide** to a

Happy Marriage

2nd Edition

13-Digit ISBN: 978-1-64643-071-0
10-Digit ISBN: 1-64643-071-9

This book may be ordered by mail from the publisher. Please include $5.99 for postage and handling. Please support your local bookseller first!

Books published by Cider Mill Press Book Publishers are available at special discounts for bulk purchases in the United States by corporations, institutions, and other organizations. For more information, please contact the publisher.

Cider Mill Press Book Publishers
"Where good books are ready for press"
PO Box 454
12 Spring Street
Kennebunkport, Maine 04046

Visit us online!
cidermillpress.com

Typography: Proxima Nova, Begum

Printed in China
1 2 3 4 5 6 7 8 9 0
First Edition

a **short guide** to a

Happy
Marriage

Sharon Gilchrest O'Neill, Ed.S.

2nd Edition

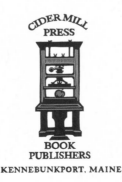

CIDER MILL
PRESS

BOOK
PUBLISHERS

KENNEBUNKPORT, MAINE

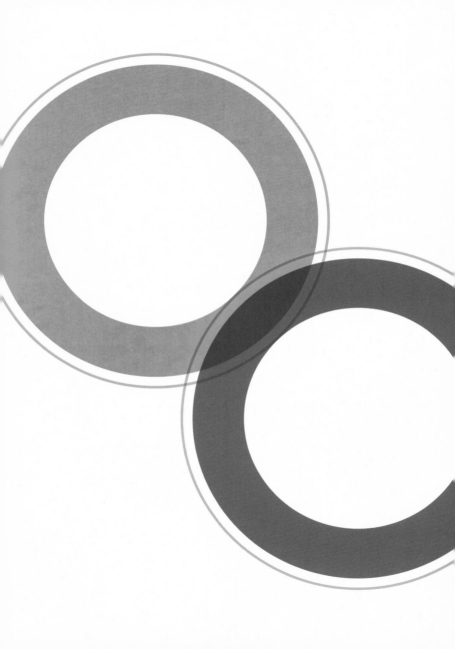

Watching and analyzing relationships

has been my passion since middle-school sleepovers with the girls, when I listened intently and gave out advice like I was Lucy from *Peanuts*, sitting behind her 5-cent psychiatric help stand. My best friends and husband would probably say that my passion has verged on the obsessive.

I carefully studied and analyzed relationships, determined to find the answers for survival: I went back to school; I became a marriage and family therapist; I read all the research, all the books; I analyzed endlessly.

Over the years, on an almost daily basis, I have been called upon to think quite seriously about the institution of marriage—its comforts and its horrors, its sensibilities and its complexities. The complexities can be so convoluted and taxing at times that many good people simply give up on marriage altogether.

So, what do I think about marriage now?

If there is any mystery about the complexity of marriage, it is about how we get there in the first place.

It is about a leap of faith that one human being makes hand-in-hand with another human being.

Well, I believe in it more than ever. Although the complexities of a relationship may feel overwhelming, the answers really are quite basic. They are about behaviors we can count on—absolute, unconditional, simple daily behaviors.

If there is any mystery about the complexity of marriage, it is about how we get there in the first place. It is about a leap of faith that one human being makes hand-in-hand with another human being.

If you are going to make that leap, you want to land safely. You need to know what you can count on—behaviors that are soothing, that have "leanability," that get you through the overwhelming times rather than stopping you in your tracks.

This book contains what I have come to consider essential to a successful marriage. It's not a scientific formulation built upon quantitative research; it's what I have witnessed over many years—those little behaviors that, when individually considered, are certainly not earth-shattering but over time create a sum in a marriage that is so much greater than its parts.

A client asked me one day, "Is there a critical mass of such behaviors? Is there a physics solution?" You be the judge as you read on.

If you are going to make that leap, you want to land safely.

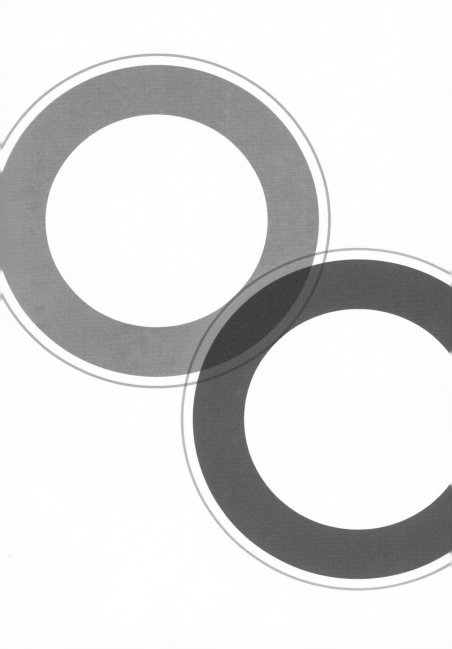

Here's a little philosophy to set the stage.

Many have conceptualized marriage as tedious, lifelong work, day in and day out. That's enough to make anyone ponder jumping ship. Marriage, to me, is better thought of as a creative work in progress. Just as the artist or writer has times when his or her work flows and all is going well, so does a marriage.

But there are the inevitable times when marriage, like work, does anything but flow. This is when you need those little behaviors you can absolutely count on for support. The experience of flow in your marriage gives you faith and hope—soak up the flow and keep it close to your heart. Just as important, keep those little behaviors going daily and going strong!

Bear in mind that marriage can only work as a team effort, as a team sport of sorts. Pump yourself up with the idea of pitting you and your spouse against the world.

Marriage, to me, is better thought of as a creative work in progress.

Celebrate your successes.

Go ahead—compare your marriage to lesser ones, brag to each other about how well you are doing together. Feel bad for others who look or act so miserable together. Celebrate your successes. Reminisce about your great team moments. Savor the memories that you will be talking about for many years to come.

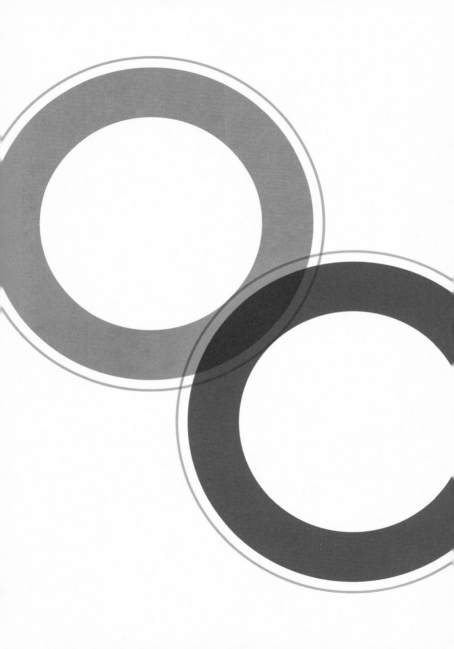

So, now,

with your newfound sense of marital team spirit, here are some little behaviors to help you along the way. Marriage means living in the same home, in the same bedroom, and in the same bed, preferably king-size. A big bed will accommodate sickness, snoring, and bedtime reading. Always be willing to splurge on practical extras like a ceiling fan above your bed and a dual-control electric blanket or a mattress pad.

No need to splurge on nightgowns or pajamas. Even if it's only your toes touching in bed as you fall into your own dreams and desires, sleeping naked is a very underrated necessity in marriage. It absolutely keeps you connected over the long haul.

On the subject of sleep, always try to go to bed together—even when you are mad at each other, even if you've been fighting all day, and even if you know that you can't make everything perfect before bedtime. Knowing you can count on ending up together, toes touching, is reassuring, soothing, and hopeful.

While on the subject of sleep and furniture, I've always thought that his-and-her chairs should

Sleeping naked is a very underrated necessity in marriage.

Knowing you can count on ending up together, toes touching, is reassuring, soothing, and hopeful.

be outlawed. Sit together on the sofa, on the floor, on a park bench—wherever you have an opportunity to be close together.

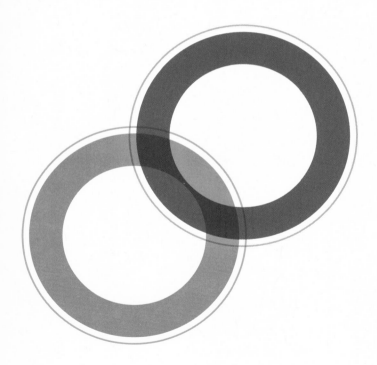

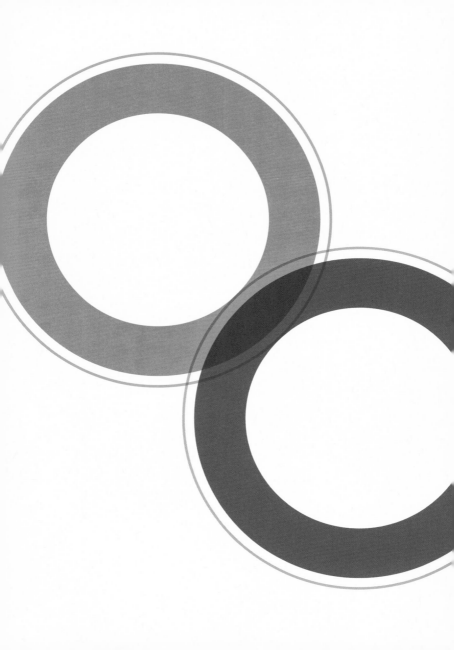

Have your own special way of connecting

during the day, at home in the evening, and over the weekend. A midday phone call, a cup of coffee or glass of wine together, a jointly home-cooked-meal night. Make it an indestructible part of the fabric of your life together. And I mean indestructible.

Only emergencies should be allowed to displace your special time together. For years, my husband and I have shared Thursday nights cooking salmon as a team, opening a nice bottle of wine, and watching TV together. Nothing takes precedence over this ritual. I can't imagine a more comforting time for the two of us—one that we've counted on and "leaned on" for years.

You may think this next behavior is not really important, but do find some hobby, sport, game, or other activity that you both can share and enjoy together. It's even better if it allows you to talk together while you do it.

Don't compartmentalize the different parts of

Don't compartmentalize the different parts of your life.

Listen to each other's agonies and ecstasies.

your life. Never completely separate your work and home lives—mix them up. Share them with your partner. Listen to each other's agonies and ecstasies.

Bring discoveries home to your partner, such as when you meet a fascinating person.

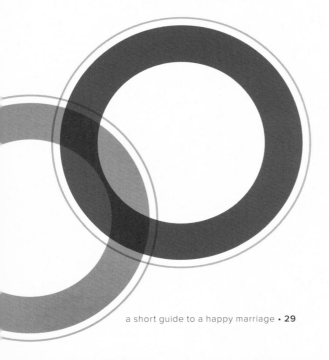

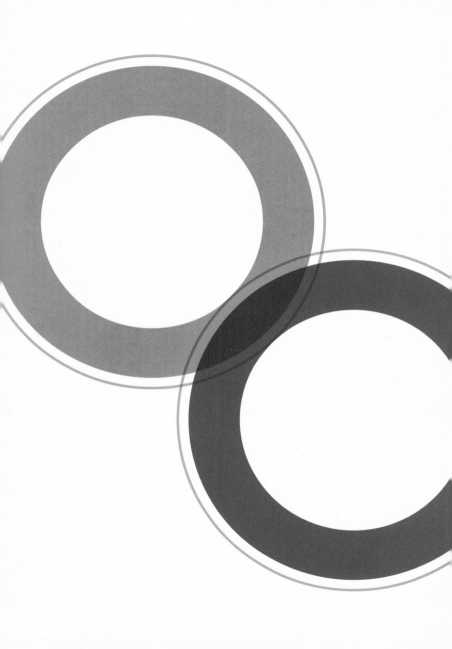

Talk, talk, talk.

It should happen every day. I like to think of touch and talk as the absolute essentials of daily married life. Talk to each other, if for only ten minutes after the chores are done and before you move on to something personally relaxing, like a TV show or a good book.

Touch, even if it's only something as quick and brief as a peck on the cheek or your toes together in bed at the end of a tiring day.

Good talk is one of the all-time great stimulants of desire. It really is an aphrodisiac.

A good marriage is always about new dreams. Things cannot stay the same; you must be able to change. You must be able to improvise, make new and different decisions, change course, and take unlikely paths. Be sure to share your dreams with each other regularly.

Good talk is one of the all-time great stimulants of desire.

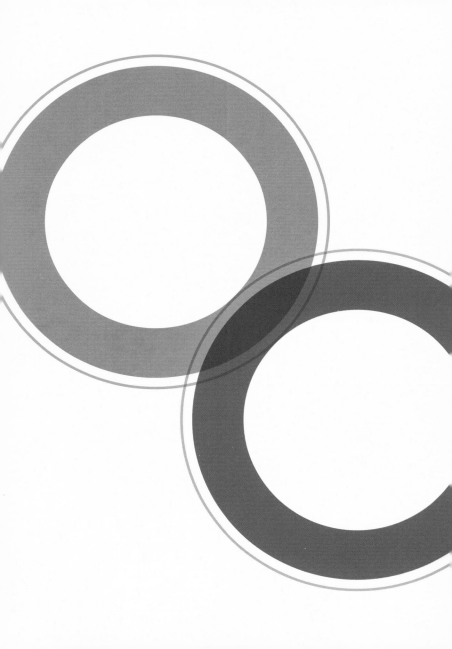

If and when children

come into the picture, be sure to constantly remind them to be loving and kind to your spouse. Set an example by letting them witness you being nicer to your spouse than to anyone else in the world. A terrific marriage is truly one of the greatest gifts you can give your children.

You must share almost everything. Your food, your kids, your money. Do not have separate bank accounts. Work through any pain you may experience from sharing; don't shove such pain under the rug.

When someone divulges a secret to you, your spouse is the one person with whom you may share it in complete confidence. This is an ultimate form of trust—someone else's secret is safe with and between the two of you. You must put your spouse first at times. If you cannot, marriage just isn't for you. To accommodate, adapt, and anticipate—these are behaviors you will often see when you watch a long-married, happy couple "at work" in their relationship.

You must share almost everything.

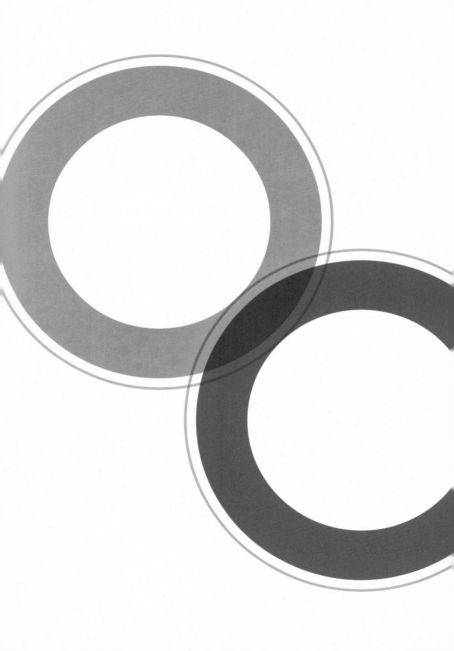

Here's an important truth

about a long, loving marriage: you will hate your spouse from time to time. That is, there will be distinct times when you really don't like your spouse—for a minute, for weeks, for months, or for some other incredibly difficult and unnerving developmental or situational period of time. This just has to be; I believe it to be truly inevitable.

The opposite will be true. That is, your spouse will hate you from time to time. This can be the more difficult part to bear. This may shake your self-esteem to its core. Hang in there.

During the times that you will inevitably experience hate—and the times that you must weather the storms, the disappointments, and the tragedies of life—you must remain a team and stay with behaviors that keep you in the flow of your marriage, remembering that your marriage is a constant work in progress.

Hang in there.

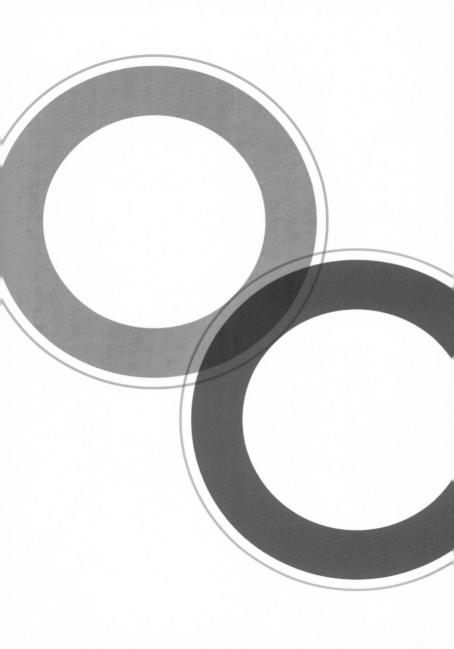

Somewhere along the way

in your marriage, do something incredibly
difficult, wonderfully giving, or deeply caring
for your spouse. Make a sacrifice. We're talking
about a once-in-a-lifetime challenge you take
on simply out of the goodness of your heart, an

exquisite gift of love, of caring, of compassion. This should be the kind of thing that others would question and perhaps not understand why you would do it. There are endless possibilities, anything from one-time events to lifelong patterns.

This might be the time to mention that quickies are crucial, always. And not just for husbands. And no faking it, ever.

Make a sacrifice. We're talking about a once-in-a-lifetime challenge you take on simply out of the goodness of your heart.

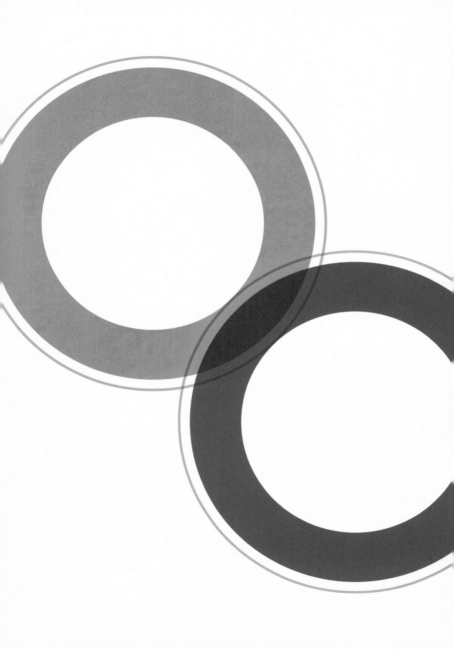

Become knowledgeable

about the number one set of skills for all couples (and families) to be proficient with: creative problem solving. There has been a lot of good stuff written about such skills—read up on it and perhaps even take classes together on creativity and problem solving. No one ever leaves my therapy office without knowing a bit more about the fun of brainstorming and creative thinking.

I have come to believe that each of us in our own unique way must hold on to a commitment to our marriage as well as to our spouse. You do have to truly believe in the institution of marriage. When the going gets tough, it may be all you can do to hang on tight to your marriage for a period of time (it's about faith and the notion of promises) and carry on with certain marriage behaviors and routines, no matter what may be rocking the boat.

In the words of author Judith Viorst: "One advantage of marriage, it seems to me, is that when you fall out of love with [your partner]...

I have come
to believe that
each of us in our
own unique way
must hold on to
a commitment
to our marriage
as well as to
our spouse.

You want to both grow in understanding the unavoidable baggage you have brought to each other.

it keeps you together until you maybe fall in again." A couple must be able to weather the storms, which are inevitable, with a belief that no one is going to walk out the door.

When a marriage is thrown a really difficult curve, such as a job loss or depression, you might be wise to find a third party to help. Do be cautious, however, of engaging in years of therapy for just one of you. You want to both grow in understanding the unavoidable baggage you have brought to each other.

I believe that you and your partner can become each other's therapists, who listen very well, really work to hear, and feed back, your thoughts and your words so you understand yourself—and each other—better than anyone else in the world. George Eliot said it so beautifully: "Oh, the comfort, the inexpressible comfort of feeling safe with a person: having neither to weigh thoughts or measure words, but to pour them out."

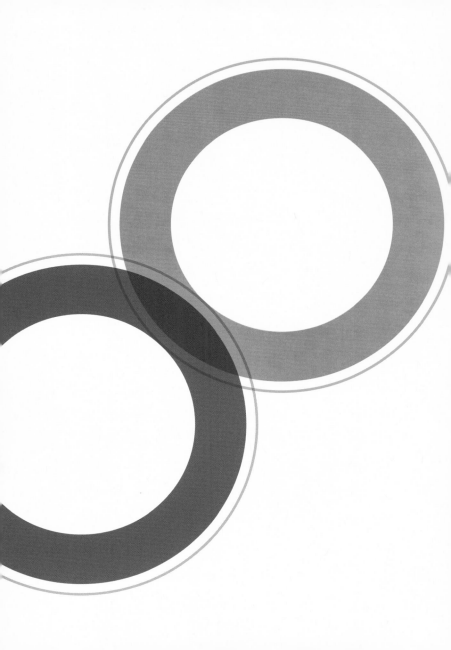

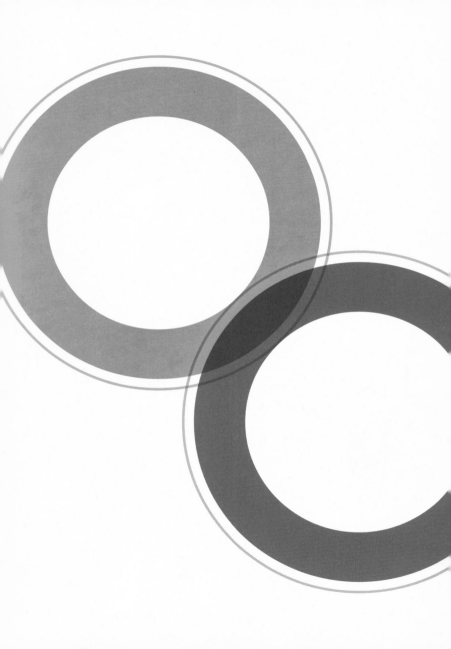

There you have it—

some behaviors to ponder, some ways to think about marriage in general, and about your marriage in particular. Know absolutely that everyone has marital problems. There are few rule books or guideposts to help us chart our course in marriage. However, knowing that you can count on certain behaviors over and over again will bring stability and safety to your marriage.

Put the behaviors in this book to good use. They are ones I have come to believe in, and they provide a place to begin that's as good as any other. I continue to be guided by these behaviors for my clients as well as for myself.

So that's it. Twenty or so behaviors to count on and to "lean on."

Do you recall the question my client posed about whether or not there is a critical mass of behaviors? I think there is. I believe in the physics of it. So try them and see what happens. As I often say to my clients:

Knowing that you can count on certain behaviors over and over again will bring stability and safety to your marriage.

They'll only get better.

"What's the worst that could happen?"

"Let's analyze your worst-case scenario."

"Will these behaviors make things worse?"

If you exercise the behaviors suggested in this book, the odds are things won't get worse. They'll only get better.

Good luck!

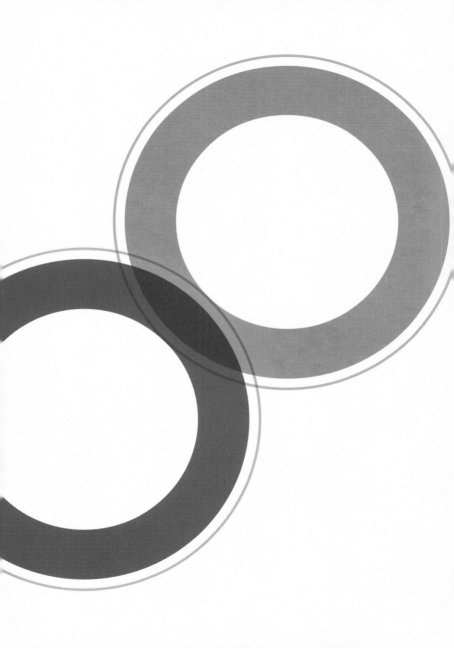

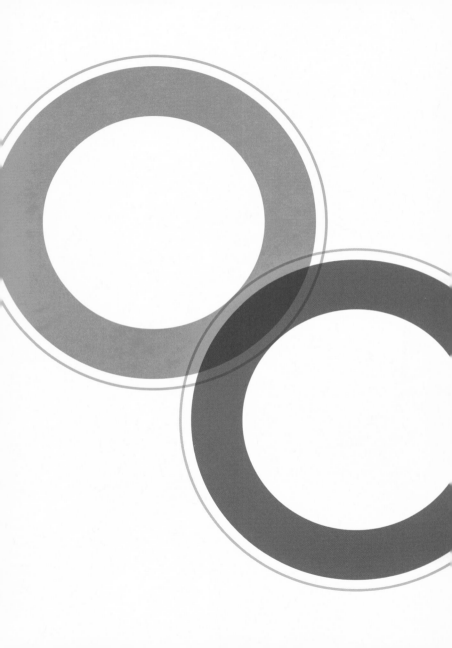

Sharon Gilchrest O'Neill, Ed.S.

is a licensed marriage and family therapist
and the author of *A Short Guide to a
Happy Divorce*, and *Sheltering Thoughts
About Loss and Grief*, and *Lur'ning: 147
Inspiring Thoughts for Learning on the Job*.
She has worked both in private practice and
the corporate setting, helping her clients to
examine assumptions, think creatively, and
build upon strengths. O'Neill holds three
degrees in psychology and is often called
on as an expert by a variety of publications,
including the *Wall Street Journal*, the *New York
Times*, the *Boston Globe*, and *HuffPost*.

About Cider Mill Press Book Publishers

Good ideas ripen with time. From seed to harvest, Cider Mill Press brings fine reading, information, and entertainment together between the covers of its creatively crafted books. Our Cider Mill bears fruit twice a year, publishing a new crop of titles each spring and fall.

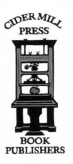

"Where Good Books Are Ready for Press"

Visit us online at
cidermillpress.com
or write to us at
PO Box 454
12 Spring St.
Kennebunkport, Maine 04046

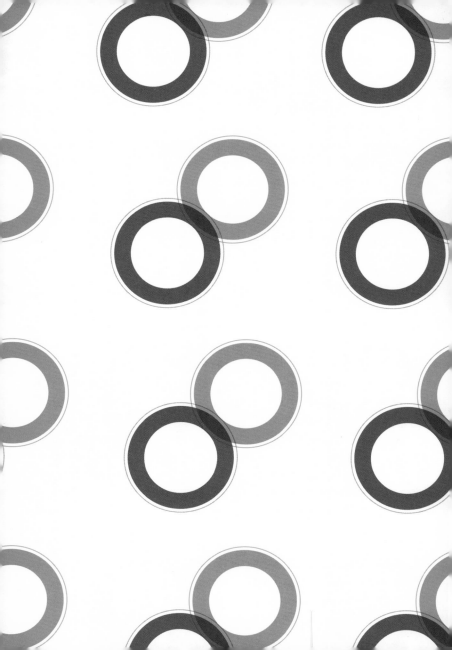

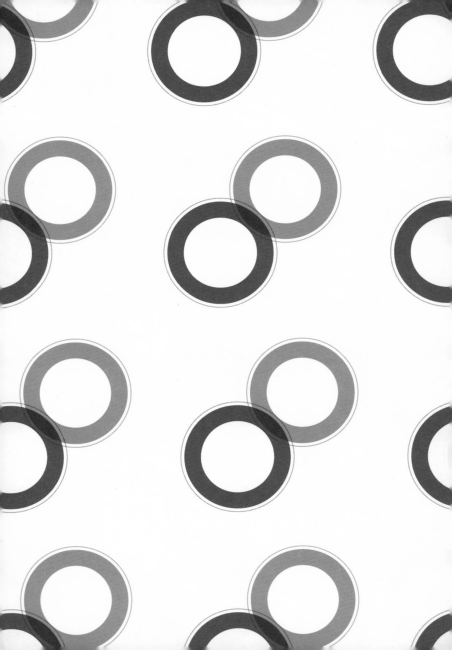